Soulful Wellness:
Integrating Body, Mind, and Spirit in Your Christian Life

Shirley Mills Dower

Contact Information: 240-630-1568
Email Address: Shirley@beinghealthwithshirley.com

Dedication

To one and only living God, my Lord and Savior Jesus Christ and the Holy Spirit for giving me the knowledge, skill and courage to write this book.

To all the people who are looking to make changes and learning how to be good stewards of their physical bodies.

To my grandchildren and great grandchildren who must learn the truth.

Acknowledgement to my daughter Katina who has been in my corner always and my spiritual daughter Carla who edited my book kicking and screaming all the way.

Thank You...

for purchasing this book. As my gift to you, please visit www.lookatshirley.com to get your Complementary Holistic Health Evaluation. A baseline for what your body is saying about your health system.

Free access to Raising Royalty Minister:

https://lddy.no/1c9g2

Also, do not forget to leave a review on Amazon.

Disclaimer

The material in this book is not intended to be psychological, medical, financial, or legal advice. Seek the appropriate counsel for those and other needs. The author is not liable for use or misuse of the information presented.

Although the author and publisher have made every effort to ensure that the information in this book was correct at press time, the author and publisher do not assume and hereby disclaim any liability to any party for any loss, damage, or disruption caused by errors or omissions, whether such errors or omissions result from negligence, accident, or any other cause.

This book is not intended as a substitute for the medical advice of physicians. The reader should regularly consult a physician in matters relating to his/her and particularly with respect to any symptoms that may require diagnosis or medical attention. The information in this book is not meant to replace proper treatment but to enhance so that you can live healthily.

So, let's begin!

Table of Contents

Letter To The Reader

Who am I?

As author of this book, I am 73 years old Christian lady and I have made a point to take charge of my health by, learning about harmful ingredients, spending time to investigate information for accuracy, and learning about the physical body requirements. I am currently active in keeping my body moving by attending a gym at least 3 times a week, in addition to walking at least 2 miles during the week. As a result of my due diligence, I am medication free, and I do not have any chronic health issues. I have been excited to tell everyone of my successful testimony.

I have been facilitator of health workshops and presentations for over 10 years passionately passing on the information that I have learned. There are those that get the health picture and others who would rather depend on medication for health issues. The bottom line is that as Christians we have a due diligence to honor our body with the right decisions. The major keys are to learn, investigate the facts, change our harmful habits, practice the new information, evaluate, and observe the results.

I want us to closely examine how preciously we have been created and what makes us different from other living things created by God.

My two main scriptures for this writing are based on Psalm 8: 4-6, "What is man that You are mindful of him, And the son of man that You visit him? For You have made him a little lower than the angels, And You have crowned him with glory and honor. You have made him to have dominion over the works of Your hands: You have put all things under his feet." (NKJV)

And 1 Corinthian 6:19-20, "Don't you realize that your body is the temple of the Holy Spirit, who lives in you and was given to you by God? You do not belong to yourself, for God bought you with a high price. So, you must honor God with your body." (NLT)

Note: Unless otherwise indicated all scriptures are taken from New Living Translation (NLT).

The purpose of this book is for us to examine how and what do we need to do to become good keepers of our physical body. We will examine the different theories about how we were created. How do you believe we were made? This book is for all human beings to examine our responsibility to being healthy. We all have the same human body and functions. Why are some of us are sick, in constant pain, take several medications a day, spent several days per week for doctor's office visits; on the other hand, some people regardless of their age are healthy, do not take daily medication, active in family and other activities outside of home?

We will examine some of the possible reasons for the differences. I pray that you will see the balance needed to thrive with your health and not simply survive. My goal is to present known facts about various aspects of our health environment. We will examine the facts in this book and investigate the truth.

This book will include a brief biology 101 of who we are, what our body needs, how our body talks to us when something is not right. We are not interested in trying to be doctors, but to know enough about our body to operate in good stewardship over our health and body.

Two quotes that come to my mind that best reflect the material in this book:

> *"Do the best you can until you know better. Then when you know better, do better."*
>
> Maya Angelou

> *"Discipline is your friend not your enemy – create good habits."*
>
> Rex Steven Spikes

Remember: Nothing changes until you change. Everything changes when you change.

My Health Ministry Affirmation:

"I honor my body with the foods that I eat, the thoughts that I think and the words that I speak."

Chapter 1: What is Man?

Man, the human being, is a magnificent creation. Have you ever studied anything about the biology of human beings? The magnificent intricate parts of the human body working together as a complete functional system. Let's discuss some of the characteristics of the human body and biological systems. Regardless of our race, color, culture, nationality, or creed, we have the same basic physical characteristics. The visually apparent aspects of appearance are what we first see about a person. Physical characteristics are said to be the defining traits or features of a person even when no other information about the person is known. How would you describe a person's physical characteristics? From your description could someone identify and pick that person out from your description? These characteristics include height, complexion, build, skin, eye color, hair, and facial features. In defining these physical characteristics, one of the first things that you will observe is a person's overall build or body type. In observation of a person, they can be described with adjectives such as short, tall, average height, extremely tall, plump, stocky, overweight, medium build, large frame, fat or skinny.

To describe a person's skin tone and complexion, several descriptive words such as dark, light, fair, rosy, olive, white, black, brown, pale, freckled, or tan can be used. In addition, for skin characteristics a person's skin appearance can be described clear, dry, age spots, oily, wrinkled, smooth, pimply, fine lines or scarred. When looking at eye colors and other eye characteristics, human eyes don't all look the same. This takes into consideration physical traits description such as the eye colors, the eye size/shapes, the eyelashes, and the eyebrows. The physical descriptions of eye colors such as blue, green, black, brown, or hazel; of eye size/shapes such as small, large, wide, slanted, close-set, or deep-set; of eyebrows such as bushy, thin, sparse, sculpted, or dark; of eyelashes such as long, short dark or light are all unique.

Next, as a person looks further at other facial features such descriptions of the nose, the cheekbones, the cheeks, the lips, and the face shape, a person can use descriptive terms such for the nose as being short, narrow, broad, long, pert or snub; for the cheekbones being high, sunken, chubby, or rosy; for the face shape being long, heart-shaped, round, oval, or thin; for the lips being thin, full, pink, red or pouty.

Lastly the physical characteristics of a person's hair further describes a person's appearance. This would include description of the hair's color, texture, shape, and length such as the colors blond, auburn, brown, black, grey, white; texture such as curly, frizzy, wavy, greasy, or matted; lengths such as long, short, bald, or receding. As you can see there are many different characteristics that can describe a person's appearance. These describe the outer appearance of a person. How accurately can you describe a person's physical characteristics? What are the internal components of a person? As we examine the biological systems of a human being, the biological are the internal components of the human being. Our human body is working 24 hours a day every second of the day. Did you know that the human body consists of approximately twelve biological systems that carry out specific functions necessary for everyday living? However, there are five vital organs that are essential for survival.

The systems are the brain, the heart, the kidneys, the liver, and the lungs. Let's briefly discuss these five organs. We are not trying to be doctors, but we need to know enough about the body to know basic problems that may be developing. Firstly, the human brain is the body's control center, receiving and sending signals to other organs through the nervous system and through secreted hormones. The brain is responsible for our thoughts, feelings, memory storage and our general perception of the world. Next is the heart, which is responsible for moving blood, nutrients, oxygen, carbon dioxide, and hormones around the body. The kidney's job is to process two hundred quarts (50 gallons) of blood to filter out about 2 quarts of waste and water. The next system is the liver whose job is to produce about 75 percent of cholesterol utilized throughout our system, detoxifying chemicals and prescription drugs and makes protein important for blood clotting. Finally, the lungs allow us to take in vital oxygen and expel carbon dioxide in the process we call breathing; on average, an adult takes over 20,000 breaths a day. There are several other internal components that work together to keep us functional. Since this is not a biology textbook on the human body, the major emphasis is identifying some of the major components to develop a sense of appreciation of the human body. As human beings we all have the same internal components. Would you not agree that the human body is an incredible creation?

According to recent research, an average person is estimated to contain 30+ trillion human cells; the human body consists of external and internal components that make up the human being. In fact, we have just scratched the surface of the human body facts. We are learning about what makes the human body a magnificent creation. What do you believe regarding how we were created? Who or what is responsible for the creation of the human being? In the next chapter, we will explore the theory or beliefs of how human beings were created. What do you believe?

Chapter 2: What Do You Believe?

Wow! As discussed in chapter 1, the questions to ask now are where, who, how and what was the creation of our human body? Regardless of the physical characteristics, every human being is different. As we explore the magnificent creation of the human being, there are at least 2 theories/beliefs; there is a scientific and a biblical theories/belief. Let us briefly explore the two theories of the creation of the human Being; the first theory is called the evolution theory and the other theory is called the Creation theory. In examining the evolution theory, one noted that scientist or the world believe that the world began as "The Big Bang Theory". The world was formed from gas and many scientists believe that Ribonucleic acid (RNA), or something like RNA, was the first molecule on Earth to self-replicate and begin the process of evolution that led to more advanced forms of life, including human beings. In the case of human evolution, Scientist believe that the lengthy process of change by which people originated from apelike ancestors. Scientific evidence shows that the physical and behavioral traits shared by all people originated from apelike ancestors and evolved over a period of approximately six million years.

One of the well-known scientists that developed a theory concerning evolution was Charles Robert Darwin. In 1859 He published a very controversial book entitled, "On the Origin of Species." It was the first formulation of the theory of Evolution by natural selection. In his book, Darwin describes how organisms evolve over generations through the inheritance of physical or behavioral trails. According to the theory the premise that within a population, there is variation in traits to help the species to adapt to environment changes that will help them survive and have more offspring. In respect of the human being, the theory is that there was an evolutionary divergence between the lineages of humans and the great apes (orangutans, chimpanzees, bonobos, and gorillas) in African continent 8-5 million years ago. The theory continues that as conditions and environment changed the ape developed into the human being due to need for survival. According to the evolution theory, as the weather climate changed the ape developed a sense to protect their selves from the elements and started living in caves; to accomplish this, there was a development of physical changes including brain sizes, facial shape, the ability to walk on two legs, the ability to create tools, and the ability to talk and reason. Thus, over millions of years, human beings changed from ape like characteristics and behavior. My concern regarding this theory is that both human beings and different forms of apelike animals still exist. There still seems to be a vast physical and behavioral difference between the apes and the human beings. Question. If human beings evolved from apes, then why are there still apes? Do you believe that human evolution started from the apes? Let's now look at the creation theory. The overall belief in the creation theory is that the world and everything in it was created by God. The reference for the creation theory is found in the Holy Bible. The Holy Bible is believed to be written over 1,900 to 3400 years old and was written by 40 different writers. The beginning of our relationship with our heavenly father started and is introduced in Genesis 1:26. "Then God said, let us make human beings in our image, to be like us." From a spiritual perception, God created all living things with an extra emphasis on the development of the human being. In Genesis 1:26 the decision was made to create man in Gods' image and then almighty God breathed in a spirit. What was God's intended relationship with man and female? To be good stewards of the things that God created including land, the environment, all the living things that has been created and one more important responsibly to love God with all our being and not have anything else above Him. There are several scriptures in the bible such as Deuteronomy 6:5 in the Old Testament and Mark 12:30 in the New Testament.

In Genesis 1:28, God blessed them and gave them the charge to multiply and reign over everything that God created. In the beginning God gave the human beings the charge and stewardship over the earth and people. As recorded in Genesis chapter 1 verses 1 to verse 25, as well as the creation of all things. God created all living things in decency and in order. First, space- earth were formed. Next a separation of time namely day and night were created. Third, a separation of the heavens from the waters of the earth were manifested. God called that space the sky. Can you imagine development of the earth? It's hard to imagine how the waters of the earth that flow in one place were created, thus creating dry ground calling the creation land and seas. Wow! We must keep in mind that these things were spoken into existence. Words are powerful! We will discuss in another chapter the power of what we think and speak. Continuing with this marvelous creation, the next every sort of vegetation which included plants and fruit bearing trees were created. What was unique was each plant and tree were created to produce seeds of their like kinds. Next, the system of time, distinguishing day from night, came into existence. The creation of sun for the day and the stars and moon for the night were spoken into existence. Do you see the order in which everything was created? After God created the right environment to support all living things, then God created fish and other living things to live in the water. He created the skies with every kind of birds and once again God's creations could produce offspring according to their kind. I believe after God created the perfect environments, He then created all living animals both on land and in the sea and in the air to thrive in those environments. There then needed to be someone to reign over all God's creation. Man was created in the image of God with a body, soul, and spirit and was above the other living things to have stewardship over the things of the earth. The question to ask now is what makes man unique and different from all other living things created by God? Let us explore some of the explanation in the next chapter. Do you get the feeling that you are special in God's eyesight? Do you believe mankind has a responsibility to care for all God creation and more importantly a responsibility to care for our own bodies?

Chapter 3: The Uniqueness of the Human Beings

As in the previous chapter, we learned that the human being was created in the likeness of God. What does that mean? What makes us different from other living things? There are at least two distinguishing characteristics that separate us from other living things. The two distinct characteristics are the ability to reason, and every human being has unique fingerprints. The first characteristic is our ability to reason. As we look at other animals created by God, the other creations function by a process to live and reproduce. If you have a pet dog or cat, observe their instincts. I have a cat named Onyx; she is a beautiful small grey cat with a unique body different from another cat I have owned. She is small with a funny body. Onyx was given to me from a litter of kittens from a friend. I don't know her breed. But as I observe her, she is quiet yet aggressive. She is well fed and spends her day licking her body to keep it clean, using the litter box and purring. She is totally dependent on me providing care for her. I keep her food and water dish full and her litter box clean. Wow! What a great life for my cat and your pets. Someone to take care of their every need! However, being totally dependent on someone could present a problem. For example, what would happen to my cat and your pets if we did not feed or take care of their basic needs? Would they live healthy and safe lives? The point of the matter is as human beings we need to use our reasoning abilities and investigate what is totally good for us.

Mankind has been given exclusively the ability to reason and make choices. Free will can be a blessing or a curse. As stated in 1 Corinthian 6:12 – "I am allowed to do anything – but not everything is good for you. And even though "I am allowed to do anything; I must not become a slave to anything." We can make choices and can reason and based on our experiences decide and reason the benefits or failure of our decision. The bible teaches us that our responsibility as believers is to work uncompromisingly as the Lord has gifted us and leads us in this life. We must fully understand that until the Lord returns there are souls to reach and ministries of every sort to be performed. We are responsible for our money, time, energy, talents, gifts, bodies, minds, and spirit. We should not invest in anything that does not in some way contribute to the work of the Lord. In James 2:26, James tells us that "As the body without the spirit is dead, so faith without deeds is dead."

Mankind is different from any other animals created by God. We have a responsibility to God and ourselves. In I Corinthians 10:31, we are told to do whatever we do to the glory of God. If we choose to not follow a healthy lifestyle, not eat in a healthy manner, practice self-control, exercise, and not care about our body, you are choosing to dishonor God and our temple. We will discuss in other chapters what this means. The other distinct characteristic is that every human being has unique fingerprints. No two people have the same fingerprint. That makes us unique and special! As we briefly examine how we come into existence, we must look at our beginnings. We started life as a union between a unique male sperm and female egg. As we developed in the womb, all our essential organs are developed at different stages. When our life's system is formed, we come into this world as unique human beings.

In the stages of life, we learn as our systems develop how to sit up, crawl, walk, feed ourselves, begin to develop what we like, recognize people in our lives, learn our names and respond when called. It is amazing how we as people navigate through the different stages of development. What do we need to support our body system? What is needed to maximize good quality of life functions to enjoy the best that life has to offer physically, mentally, and spiritually. In our next chapter, we will explore the 2 broad medical systems and their attributes and benefits provided to our body.

Chapter 4: Methodologies of Medicine and its History

When we want to maintain good health or check on health issues, where do we go for assistance? In the United States there are two primary systems of medicine, allopathic, known as Western medicine and holistic, known as Eastern medicine. Allopathic medicine focuses on treating symptoms with drugs and surgery and Holistic medicine considers the whole person, including physical, mental, and spiritual health. In terms of current statistics on the two systems, the allopathic, Western medicine is used 62% by people in the United States and the holistic, Eastern medicine is used 38%. In this chapter we will review medical history in the United States. The statistics mentioned have not always been the case in the United States.

First, let's dig deeper regarding the methodologies of the two systems. Each system will be evaluated according to their respective philosophy, approach, diagnosis, treatment, emphasis, follow-up, patient involvement, cost, and length of treatment. In terms of philosophy, Allopathic medicine focuses on treating symptoms with drugs and surgery. Allopathic medicine is divided into several specific areas of specialization according to different body areas. Family practice physicians treat people of all ages. Pediatricians treat children from birth to young adulthood. Geriatric physicians focus on caring for older adults. Allergists focus on preventing and treating allergic conditions and diseases. Dermatologists focus on treating diseases and conditions of the skin, nail, and hair. Ophthalmologists specialize in eye and vision care. Cardiologists focus on care for the cardiovascular system, Nephrologists focus on kidney care. Urologists treat conditions of the urinary tract. Neurologists treat conditions of the nerves, spine and brain. Psychiatrists treat mental health conditions, and Oncologists treat cancer and its symptoms.

Specialized surgeons, such as general surgeons, perform surgical procedures. Orthopedic surgeons specialize in treating diseases and conditions of the bones, muscles, ligaments, tendons, and joints. Cardiac surgeons perform surgeries on the heart and the major surrounding blood vessels. Anesthesiologists ensure a person's well-being before, during, and after surgery by providing the proper administration of anesthetics and developing anesthetic plans. Each type of doctor undergoes their own unique training and education. In most cases, people first see a primary care physician then are referred or recommended to the specialist. The allopathic system breaks the body down based on the body area and the appropriate specialization needed.

On the other hand, Holistic medicine looks at the body interconnected whole; Holistic medicine considers the whole person, including physical, mental, and spiritual. The doctors included in holistic medicine includes naturopathic doctors who believe that the body, mind, and spirit are all connected as a unified whole. Acupuncturist are trained in ancient Chinese medicine inserting needles to relieve blockages of energy. Chiropractors use hand techniques to manipulate the bone structure of patients, specifically the spine. Homeopathies utilize plants and minerals in the treatment of patients. These two systems of medicine are greatly debated in the medical field. When we compare the two systems, Allopathic medicine focuses on treating symptoms and diagnosis of the problem using laboratory test and medical imaging. Holistic medicine also uses lab tests and imaging, in addition to interviewing patients regarding lifestyle, diet and emotions.

Let's compare the treatment for the two systems, allopathic medicine primarily uses drugs and surgery, while holistic medical treatment uses natural remedies, such as nutrition, herbs, acupuncture, and massage. The emphasis of allopathic medicine emphasizes <u>cure of symptoms</u>, while holistic medicine emphasizes <u>prevention</u>. Simply put, allopathic medicine treats the disease and holistic medicine treats the individual.

In terms of follow-up allopathic medicine may require follow-up appointments, while holistic medicine encourages self-care and lifestyle changes based on providing education to the patients. Allopathic medical treatments often ignore social, emotional, and spiritual factors, while holistic medical treatments consider those factors. Another crucial factor is that allopathic medicine may exclude the patient in the treatment process, while holistic medical treatment encourages patient participation and involves educating the patient regarding the treatment process. In specialization, allopathic medicine often involves many specialists, while holistic medicine may involve a general practitioner or holistic healthcare provider.

The length of treatment for allopathic medicine may require short term treatment by quieting the symptoms the body is trying to tell us while the condition remains, while Holistic medicine often involves longer-term lifestyle changes through education and practice. The overall focus for Allopathic medicine focuses on specific diseases and conditions, while holistic medicine focuses on overall health and wellness of the individual. Regarding cost, Allopathic medicine is usually covered by health insurance, while Holistic medicine is self-pay. A brief history of why the difference between coverage components of the two systems will be discussed in the next section.

Both Allopathic and Holistic doctors must earn a 4-year degree in a science or related field. Allopathic doctors must complete an allopathic medical program. Holistic doctors must complete a four-year, graduate-level naturopathic medical school and are educated in all the same basic sciences as an allopathic doctor. However, holistic doctors must study holistic nontoxic approaches to therapy with a strong emphasis on disease prevention and optimizing wellness. There are vast differences between the two systems of medicine. Both are healthcare options but have different methodologies. Let's briefly discuss the history of medicine in America to delve into the changes in medicine in America throughout the years.

In the early 1900, natural and herbal medicines were very popular in America. There were a variety of doctors and healing modalities in America. There was not a monopoly of all the different types of healthcare disciplines. The question now is why the change in healthcare and changes in the monopoly of one health discipline over another? Let's review recorded historical events in America. What changed in the western medicine business story? John D. Rockefeller (1839-1937) is considered the wealthiest American of all time. Reviewing history Rockefeller is most famous for securing a monopoly in America's oil market.

During the turn of the 20th century, Rockefeller controlled 90% of all petroleum refineries in America through ownership of the Standard Oil Corporation. During the same era scientists were doing ground-breaking work to understanding the basic mechanics of life and human health. As Rockefeller wanted to benefit from the medical industry, his first move with his vast wealth was to purchase part of the German pharmaceutical company I.G. Farben. Now that he controlled a drug manufacturing company, his plan was to eliminate the competition. However, he realized that there were multiple medical schools in America who first line of treatment was not prescription drugs. To eliminate the competition for non-drug or reduced drug treatment, he hired a contractor named Abraham Flexner to investigate medical practices in America. He then submitted a report, Flexner Report, to Congress in 1910. The summary of the report stated that there were too many doctors and medical schools in America, and that all natural healing modalities which had existed for hundreds of years were unscientific and quackery. This report called for the standardization of medical education, whereby only the American Medical Association would be allowed to grant medical school licensure in America. Based on the report, congress acted upon the Flexner's recommendation and changed laws related to medical practice. As a result, allopathic medicine became the standard modality.

With the new laws in place, Rockefeller teamed up with Andrew Carnegie who was also a billionaire in the steel industry. With their wealth and political power, they started funding medical schools all over America on the strict conditions that they only taught allopathic medicine. Through their power of their huge "grants", this powerful team completely changed the previous curricula of the medical schools removing any mention of the healing power of herbs or natural treatments, teaching on diet and other natural non-drug treatments.

Rockefeller and Carnegie are known as plutocrats and oligarchy, a person whose power <u>derives</u> from their wealth and a small group of people having control of a country, organization, or institution. In this case, they controlled the medical institution. After successfully removing traditional medicine from medical schools, Rockefeller made sure to secure his monopoly on the medical industry by discrediting and demonizing through the newspapers and other media of that time. Even some doctors were jailed for using natural medicine treatments. In a very short time, medical colleges were all homogenized. All the students were taught the same allopathic system and medicine was then defined as a process of prescribing patented drugs.

Wow, money talks! In summary, the diligent work of Rockefeller and Carnegie crushed the holistic system and created the monopoly of the allopathic medicine system that rules today. With their influence in the political world, they also established that healthcare insurance would not approve holistic medicine thus anyone wanting to use holistic medicine would have to self-pay for the treatment. This gave rise to the current medical system we see today. As a result, medical students are taught the same thing- to use petrochemicals in the form of drugs to mask the symptoms. What could possibly go wrong with this process? Well, this is not what "Health Care" is supposed to be all about. This should truly be called "Sick Care". Unfortunately, doctors today learn little to nothing about nutrition, holistic practices, and natural medicine. Could this be why our nation's health is in crisis? Not only is the "Health Care" system broken, but the focus is on disease management not disease prevention and doctors have become glorified drug pushers/dealers for the pharmaceutical companies. I invite you to investigate the history of the United States medical system for yourself. We must be cautious in what we hear and believe and investigate to ensure we are receiving optimal care.

Another matter of concern to the healthcare system, was in 1939 a "Drug Trust" alliance was formed by the Rockefeller empire and the German chemical company I.G. Farben (Bayer). After World War II, I.G. Farben was dismantled but later emerged as separate corporations within the alliance. Well-known companies included General Mills, Kellogg, Nestle, Bristol-Myers Squibb, Procter and Gamble, Roche, and Hoechst (Sanofi-Aventis). This alliance with Chase Manhattan Bank (now JP Morgan Chase), owns over half of the pharmaceutical interests in the United States. It is the largest drug manufacturing merger in the world. When Jesus sent out the disciples, he gave them specific instruction on dealing with the world. In Matthew 10:16, His instructions were," look, I am sending you out as sheep among wolves. So be as shrewd as snakes and harmless as doves." Chapter 5 introduces factors that have affected our health and healthcare.

Chapter 5: Environmental Changes that Affect Our Health?

In the previous chapter, we discussed how the healthcare system was completely changed in 1910 by the Flexner Report. The Flexner Report examined medical education and reform was suggested for medical colleges to include increasing standards, closing schools that could not maintain or update their facilities and partnering with hospitals for clinical training. The Flexner Report transformed the nature of medical education in America with a resulting elimination of proprietary traditional schools and the establishment of the Allopathic model as the gold standard of medical training. This effort was done by two plutocrats namely John Rockefeller and Andrew Carnegie. There have been environmental changes that also have tremendous impact on our food sources in America. The two main areas are Senate Document 264 and the Green Revolution project.

Senate Document 264 was a report presented to congress in 1936 addressing the poor mineral composition of the soil needed for the farming of our food and the minerals need for healthy human consumption and dietary needs. Rex Beach wrote an article titled, "Modern Miracle Men" which reported on Dr. Charles Northen who stopped his medical work and shifted to agriculture because he felt he could help many more people by improving their diets. Dr. Northen found after analyzing the soil in our farmlands, that American soil lacked the necessary minerals required for effective growth of our food and the minerals needed for healthy diets. During his practice, Dr. Northen specialized in treating stomach diseases and nutritional disorders. He began seeing an increase of his patients with degenerative diseases and found no solution in sight. Dr. Northen was the first man in this field of research, to demonstrate that most human foods grown were poor in minerals and that their proportions were not balanced across America's farmlands. For example, a vegetable or fruit grown on one farm in the United States would have different nutritional value than fruit or vegetables grown in another part of the country. The implication is poor soil has major impact on the health of the individuals that consume food especially if the soil does not have the necessary minerals.

According to the article, Dr. Northen reported a 10-year test with rats proving that by withholding calcium they can be bred down to a third the size of those fed with an adequate amount of that minerals. It was also found that the rat's intelligence could be changed by mineral feeding as readily as can their size, bone structure, and their general health. In addition, rats, guinea pigs, and other animals can be fed into a diseased condition and out again by controlling only the minerals in their food. If you place a number of these little animals inside a maze after starving some of them in a certain mineral element the starved ones will be unable to find their way out. However, the non-starving animals will have little or no difficulty in getting out. Their dispositions can be altered by mineral feeding. Animals can be made aggressive and combative and even be turned into cannibals and be made to devour each other based on their mineral consumption.

In terms of human beings, many children are "delayed" merely because they are deficient in magnesium and other vital minerals. We punish them for our failure to feed them properly. Northen further stated that our physical well-being is more directly dependent upon the minerals we take into our systems than upon calories or vitamins or the precise proportions of starch, protein, or carbohydrates we consume. His research and other researchers concluded that it is now agreed that at least 16 mineral elements are indispensable for normal nutrition, and several more are always found in small amounts in the body, although their precise physiological role has not been determined. Calcium, phosphorus, and iron are perhaps the most important of the indispensable salts. Calcium is the dominant nerve controller. Calcium powerfully affects the cell formation of all living things and regulates nerve action. Calcium governs contractility of the muscles and the rhythmic beat of the heart. It also coordinates the other mineral elements and corrects disturbances made by them. It works in the sunlight. Vitamin D is its buddy.

As a result of Dr. Northen research finding, Senate Document 264 of 1936 was presented to congress. The reported basically indicated that:

- "Fruits and vegetables and grains ... are starving us--no matter how much of them we eat! "

- "No man of today can eat enough fruits and vegetables to supply his stomach with the mineral salts he requires "

- "99% of the American people are deficient in these minerals ... Any upset of the balance ... and we sicken, suffer, and shorten our lives. "

- " Lacking minerals, vitamins are useless."

His bottom line: "It is simpler to cure sick soils than sick people." Which shall WE choose? "Sick soils mean sick plants, sick animals, and sick people."

This was report in 1936 to congress; however, no action was taken due to amount of cost to correct the situation and it was during the inter-war period. The eminent authority and others ridicule Dr. Northen and stated that nutrition and minerals had nothing to do with people being sick. **If you remember nutrition and food were not included in the allopathic medical studies.**

The second area of concern regarding our environmental practices is the Green Revolution. Due to world hunger, the Green Revolution was developed around 1960. Dr. Norman Borlaug was an American agronomist known as the "father of the Green Revolution". The Green Revolution led to high productivity of crops through adapted measures, such as:

1) increasing the areas being farmed,

2) double cropping, which includes planting two crops rather than one, annually,

3) adoption of High Yield Varieties (HYV) of seeds,

4) highly increased use of inorganic fertilizers and pesticides,

5) improved irrigation facilities, and

6) improved farm implements and crop protection measures

To continue using Green Revolution technologies to produce more food for a growing population worldwide, the Rockefeller Foundation and the Ford Foundation, as well as many government agencies around the world funded increased research. A new variety of grains were created that included new seeds that had pesticides that would kill the insect's destruction of the crops. But if the new seeds had pesticides repellants what would happen to us as human beings when we continually consume the foods of grains of these crops?

According to history, Norman Borlaug who was awarded the Nobel Peace Prize in 1970 was credited with saving at least a billion lives from starvation based on his efforts of breeding varieties of grains. The Green Revolution led initiatives that "involved the development of high-yielding varieties of cereal grains which are wheat, corn and rice, distribution of hybridized seeds, synthetic fertilizers, and pesticides to farmers. He pioneered a new "improved" species of semi-dwarf wheat that, together with complimenting fertilizers and pesticides, increased yield spectacularly. This amazing new farming technology was propagated around the world by companies like Dupont and Monsanto, while mid-20th-century humanity applauded the end of hunger. The Green Revolution was about solving world hunger, but we're now discovering some unintended consequences. Gluten is a protein found in many grains, including wheat, barley, and rye. It's common in foods such as bread, pasta, pizza, and cereal. Gluten provides no essential nutrients. People with celiac disease have an immune reaction that is triggered by eating gluten. Symptoms of gluten problems in which digestive symptoms may come in the form of diarrhea, constipation, abdominal pain, reflux, gas, or even vomiting. Meanwhile, individuals may also experience other symptoms, including fatigue, joint pain, brain fog, and even bouts of depression due to gluten. What we need to ensure is that our health is thriving and not just surviving. In the next chapter, we will discuss how to be conquerors.

Chapter 6: Thriving not just Surviving

As we discussed in the previous chapter, there are theories regarding how we were created. This book is focused on the creation theory that God created everything and man was God's prize creation. As stated in Genesis 1:26, we were created in God's image. In addition, in Genesis 1:28, "God blessed them and said "Be fruitful and multiply fill the earth and govern it. Reign over the fish in the sea, the birds in the sky, and all the animals that scurry along the ground. This is one of the purposes of man is to be steward and maintain stewardship of the earth. Stewardship is defined as the conducting, supervising, or managing of something especially the careful and responsible management of something entrusted to one's care. This includes property, money, time, talents, relationships, and our bodies. One of the main scriptures in the holy Bible which are the foundational scriptures for my health ministry is I Corinthian 6: 19-20. "Don't you realize that your body is the temple of the Holy Spirit, who lives in you and was given to you by God? You do not belong to yourself. For God bought you with a high price. So, you must honor God with your body. "How do we obey that command?

We first must evaluate our physical blindness. What do you mean physical blindness? **I am glad you asked.**

First, we must know the basics of what our wonderful body requires to thrive and be ultimately healthy. We discussed in the last chapter how two powerful plutocrats totally monopolized the healthcare system namely Rockefeller and Carnegie, reducing our equal health options. Let's examine some scriptures that can affect how we view things and how we as Christians can be misled. It is also important to understand that words are powerful, and the Word of God is extremely powerful. Providing biblical evidence of how God wanted us as His creation to treat our bodies, I believe is important. Let's look at some of the scriptures:

- 1 Corinthian 3:16 – 19 states "Don't you realize that all of you together are the temple of God and that the Spirit of God lives in you? God will destroy anyone who destroys this temple. For God's temple is holy, and you are that temple. Stop deceiving yourselves. If you think you are wise by this world's standards, you need to become a fool to be truly wise. For the wisdom of this world is foolishness to God. As the Scriptures say, He traps the wise in the snare of their own cleverness."

- Romans 12: 1- 2 states "And so, dear brother and sisters, I plead with you to give your bodies to God because of all he has done for you. Let them be a living and holy sacrifice – the kind he will find acceptable. This is truly the way to worship him. Don't copy the behavior and customs of this world, but let God transform you into a new person by changing the way you think. Then you will learn to know God's will for you, which is good, pleasing, and perfect."

- In 1 Corinthian 6:12 the Apostle Paul states, "I am allowed to do anything – but not everything is good for you. And even though "I am allowed to do anything; I must not become a slave to anything." Our free will is a giant in our life which can be a blessing or a curse. We talk and pray about evil principalities but my brother and sister, the giant that we face every day, maybe ourselves and our free will.

We must remember! Be diligent in learning and investigating foods and our lifestyles. It could mean the difference between thriving and just surviving. Let's first have a brief human biology 101. As we examine human biological systems, the biological are the internal components of the human being. Our human bodies are working 24 hours a day every second of the day. The adult human body contains 213 bones; approximately 100 trillion cells; 30 trillion red blood cells in 60,000 miles of blood vessels; and 2 million sweat glands on its surface. The lungs are composed of 700 million cells. If the heartbeats for a single day were concentrated into one huge throb of vital power, it would be sufficient to throw a ton of iron 120 feet into the air. Massive right? As stated previously, did you know that the human body consists of approximately 12 biological systems that carry out specific functions necessary for everyday living? However, there are five vital organs that are essential for survival. The systems are the brain, the heart, kidneys, liver, and the lungs. Let's briefly discuss each organ. We are not doctors, but we need to know enough about the body to understand basic problems that may be developing.

First, the human brain is the body's control center, receiving and sending signals to other organs through the nervous system and through secreted hormones. The brain is responsible for our thoughts, feelings, memory storage and our general perception of the world. Next is the heart responsible for moving blood, nutrients, oxygen, carbon dioxide, and hormones around the body. The kidney's job is to process 200 quarts (50 gallons) of blood to filter out about 2 quarts of waste and water. The next system is the liver whose job is to produce about 75 percent of cholesterol utilize throughout our system, detoxifying chemicals and prescription drugs and makes protein important for blood clotting. Finally, the lungs allow us to take in vital oxygen and expel carbon dioxide in the process we call breathing; on average, an adult takes over 20,000 breaths a day. There are several other internal components that work together to keep us functional. Since this is not a biology textbook on the human body, the major emphasis is identifying some of the major components to develop a sense of appreciation of the human body. Would you not agree that the human body is an incredible creation? According to recent research, an average person is estimated to contain 30+ trillion human cells. The human body consists of external and internal components that makes up the human body. In fact, we have just scratched the surface about the human body. We are learning about what makes the human body a magnificent creation. The key point is knowing the basic of our bodily systems and what is right for our body is critical. **Remember we can do better when we know better.**

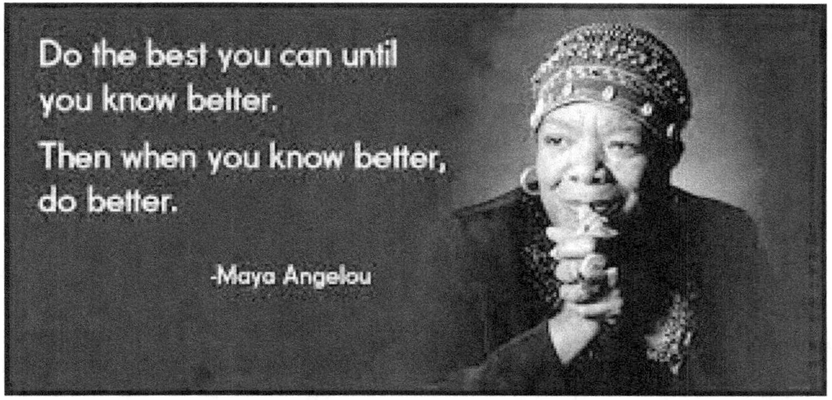

By now it should be clear that the body's cellular makeup provides structure and function for the human body. Take the health IQ quiz on the next page and test your health awareness.

Exercise 1

Your Health IQ Quiz

Test Yourself: *Answer the following questions. See Appendix 1 for the correct answer.*

1. What does GMO stand for? *Circle one answer*
   a. Good Mouth Odor   c. Genetic Made Organ
   b. Good Mental Output   d. Genetic Modified Organism

2. What is the hardest substance or part of your body?

   ____

3. GMO is healthy for our body? ☐ True ☐ False

4. What is your body's largest organ? _________________

5. Hair and nails are made of _______________________

6. If we eat the right healthy foods, we will have the required minerals and vitamins needed to stay healthy?

   ☐ True ☐ False

The importance of nutrients and their role in the body

What is nutrition? Nutrients are the nourishing substances in food that are essential for the growth, development, and maintenance of body functions. Essential meaning that if a nutrient is not present, aspects of function and therefore human health decline." (Jones, D.S. (editor) (2006). Textbook of Functional Medicine. Gig Harbor, Washington: Institute for Functional Medicine.)

The subject of nutrition, as we think of it today, is not explicitly mentioned in the Bible—that is, the Bible doesn't talk about calories and the balance of fat, protein, and carbohydrates a person needs. Neither does it mention GMOs or the benefits of eating whole foods versus processed food. The production of food had not yet been industrialized at the time the Holy Bible was written. As indicated in 3 John 1:2, "Dear friend, I hope all is well with you and that you may be in good health, as it goes well with your soul." Furthermore, from a holistic and biological standpoint the elements in food, which vitamins and minerals were vital for optimal health and wellness, and how they aid the human body were not yet established. However, from biblical principles we can deduce that it is beneficial and even morally right to emphasize a healthy diet containing all the essential nutrients.

The Bible encourages us to care for our bodies, and good nutrition is naturally part of that. God cares about man's physical comfort and well-being. As indicated in 1

Corinthians 6: 18-20, Paul argues that, since a believer's body is a temple of the Holy Spirit, he should flee sexually immorality, which harms the body that was bought by Christ's blood. This argument can be carried over to other issues, including drug and alcohol abuse and how we eat food. Food is fuel. It is not meant to be used purely for pleasure, or we could eat nothing but chocolate and cheese pizza and be healthy. Food is meant for nutrition and good health. We should strive to eat to live not live to eat. Our bodies can be considered machines that carry us from place to place as we conduct the work God has planned for us. For we are God's masterpiece. He has created us anew in Christ Jesus, so we can do the good things He planned for us long ago. (Ephesians 2:10). An unhealthy body will make us slow, lethargic, and prone to illness and injury. Good nutrition is critical for proper brain function and hormonal balance. Eating the right food contributes highly to our ability to think clearly and to our overall quality of life. Therefore, good nutrition helps support our service for the Lord.

God provides food to us, as He does to the creatures of the animal kingdom (Psalm 147:9; 104:27; 136:25). The earth has been created to produce foods that are full of vitamins and minerals and amino acids that the body needs to survive and be healthy. Food is a gift from God; it is His provision. Why do whole, raw, unprocessed foods contain the most nutrition? Because they come right from God's hand. God tells us in 1 Corinthians 6: 19-20 that our body is the temple of the Holy Spirit which is an honor in stewardship of our physical body. In 1 Corinthians 10:31, we are told to do whatever we do to the glory of God. ... If you choose to not follow a healthy lifestyle, not eat in a healthy manner, not practice self-control, exercise, and or care about your body, you are choosing to not honor God. Hebrew 4:12 indicates, the word of God is alive and powerful. It is sharper than the sharpest two-edged sword, cutting between soul and spirit, between joint and marrow. It exposes our innermost thoughts and desires. Nothing in all creation is hidden from God. Everything is naked and exposed before his eyes, and He is the one to whom we are accountable. How do we know what is good and healthy to eat and support our body? The key to that is to educate ourselves on the basic elements of what we consume, especially our growing children. It is vital that children develop into healthy adults equipped with good eating habits which they will learn from what we do and speak. The bottom line is that we do better when we know better through educating ourselves and investigating facts given to us. Learn to dig deeper into your health. Don't just take things at face value. Ask probing questions. Don't feel uncomfortable asking who, what when, where or why as it relates to your body or your health.

Let's get started on some nutrients and nutrition facts.

Did you know that you are what you eat! Every 28 days our skin replaces itself. Are there times while bathing when there appears to be what looks to dirt on your skin? However, is it our skin shedding for new skin. Your liver is replaced every 5 months, and your bones every 10 years. Your body makes new cells from the food you eat. What you literally eat becomes you. The bottom line is that you have a choice of what you are made of. The funny cartoon below illustrates this point. It's a squirrel, and he is told that he is what he eats. And he said, "When I learned you are what you eat. I realized I was nuts." **Get it!!**

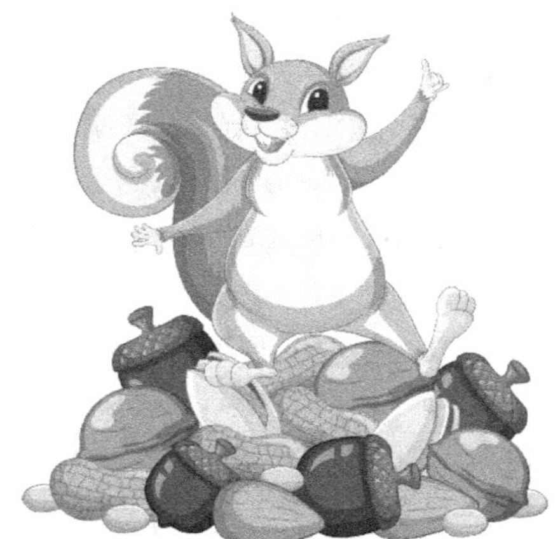

You are what you eat!

The Federal Drug Administration (FDA) has provided a list of at least 90 vitamins and minerals that our body require daily to function. Our body needs all three macronutrients which are proteins, carbs, and fats. In addition, our body needs micronutrients which are vitamins and minerals. Recall in Chapter 5, Senate Document 264 provided a wealth of information to Congress regarding how soil used to grow food was depleted of all the minerals needed to support our food, animals and people. That report was sent to Congress over eighty years ago and if the problem was not corrected and properly addressed then we must investigate and find an alternative solution. Let's examine some factors we have control over. We should learn to properly read food labels, understand which ingredients may be harmful to our health, dangers of processed foods, the impact of sugar on the body, and understand what healthy foods are and the benefits of eating whole foods.

Reading food labels

Food labels of some form existed back in ancient times. In 1850, food labels began to appear on food after the death of the 12th President of the United States Zachary Taylor from foodborne illness. About 12 years later in 1862, President Abraham Lincoln created the United States Department of Agriculture (USDA)

Other events that led to food labeling as it exists today are:

- In 1906, the Pure Food and Drug Act and the Meat Inspection Act was passed. The first federal law which prohibits false or misleading statements.

- In 1913, the Could Amendment was added to requiring contents to be plainly marked on the outside food package.

- In 1938, The Food, Drug, and Cosmetic Act took effect, requiring any artificial flavoring, coloring or chemical preservative to be listed on food labels.

- In 1967, the Fair Packaging and Labeling Act required ingredients to be listed in descending order of quantity.

- In 1990, the Nutrition Labeling and Education Act empowered consumers to make informed decisions regarding their health and wellness.

- In 2020, there was a proposal for a new nutrition label.

Let's go back for a moment and define what a food label is. Food labels provide information to consumers about ingredients, and the nutritional composition of packaged food for sale. Labels may also contain information about the conditions under which the food was produced. In addition, a Nutrition Facts label is found on the packaging which lists the nutritional content, the serving size, and the calories for a recommended serving of the food product. Finally, food labels are a legal requirement, and are important for many reasons. Food labels provide consumers with information that help them make informed choices about the food they purchase. Food labels also provide information regarding how to safely store food and when to consume it by providing an expiration date. These factors help reduce food wastage.

Below is an example of a food label:

Nutrition Facts
Serving Size 2/3 cup (55g)
Servings Per Container About 8

Amount Per Serving

Calories 230	Calories from Fat 72

	% Daily Value*
Total Fat 8g	12%
Saturated Fat 1g	5%
Trans Fat 0g	
Cholesterol 0mg	0%
Sodium 160mg	7%
Total Carbohydrate 37g	12%
Dietary Fiber 4g	16%
Sugars 1g	
Protein 3g	

Vitamin A	10%
Vitamin C	8%

Nutrition Facts
8 servings per container
Serving size 2/3 cup (55g)

Amount per serving
Calories 230

	% Daily Value*
Total Fat 8g	10%
Saturated Fat 1g	5%
Trans Fat 0g	
Cholesterol 0mg	0%
Sodium 160mg	7%
Total Carbohydrate 37g	13%
Dietary Fiber 4g	14%
Total Sugars 12g	
Includes 10g Added Sugars	20%
Protein 3g	

The next step is to investigate reading the food labels and identify harmful food additives. In being good stewards of our physical bodies, we must learn about ingredients that are harmful to our health and that cause continued chronic diseases.

Let's talk about food additives and why food and color ingredients are added to food:

- Food additives and food colors are used to maintain or improve safety and freshness and preserve slow product spoilage.

- Help to control contamination and improve or maintain nutritional value of vitamins and minerals (and fiber).

- Restore loss due to diet or loss in processing.

- Improve taste, texture and appearance such as spices, natural and artificial flavors, and sweeteners added to enhance taste.

The types of food additives are:

- Anti-caking agents - stop ingredients from becoming lumpy.

- Sorbic acids/ benzoic acid - prevent foods from oxidizing or going rancid.

- Artificial sweeteners - increase the sweetness.

- Emulsifiers - stop fats from clotting together.

- Food acids - maintain the right acid level.

- Colors - enhance or add color and

- Humectants - keep foods moist.

Here is a list of additives and other harmful ingredients found on food labels. Investigate for yourself to evaluate the harm that they do to the body. The questions to ask is if your current foods contain any of these harmful ingredients and how is your body functioning and feeling?

- Sodium nitrates/nitrites- process meats

- Hydrogenated oils, aka trans-fat - fried foods and bakery products

- Sugar in all its forms – such as corn syrup, dextrose sucrose

- Artificial flavors and colors – not made from food products and are not meant to go in the body

- Artificial sweeteners - sucralose, aspartame, saccharin

- Oils: Corn, vegetable, soybean - These oils contain wrong balance the omega-6 fats than most other oils

- Enriched wheat - This flour has been processed to remove the bran and endosperm of the wheat grain

- Carrageenan - It is used to thicken foods and is commonly found in low-fat dairy products and dairy alternatives

- Potassium or sodium benzoate - preservatives added to soft drinks and juices - inhibit the growth of mold, bacteria, and yeast

- Bisphenol A, aka BPA - found in the epoxy resin lining aluminum cans, the lining of some glass jar lids

Wow! These are some powerful ingredients that we should avoid at all costs.

Dangers of processed foods

Did you know that processed foods can be often harmful to our health. We have become such a convenience generation and we want everything quick and easy. Let's discuss what processed foods are.

According to the **United States Department of Agriculture (USDA)**, processed foods are:

Any raw agricultural commodities that have been washed, cleaned, milled, cut, chopped, heated, pasteurized, blanched, cooked, canned, frozen, dried, dehydrated, mixed or packaged. Ready-to-eat foods, such as crackers, chips, and deli meat, are more heavily processed. The most heavily processed foods often are frozen or premade meals, including frozen pizza and microwaveable dinners.

Anything done that alters food natural state. This may include adding preservatives, flavors, nutrients and other food additives, or substances approved for use in food products, such as salt, sugars, and fats. This basically means that anything that we eat that we didn't prepare ourselves is a processed food. When was the last time you prepared mashed potatoes from potatoes or other ingredients, mashed, and served from scratch? In today's busy environment we would either purchase a box of potatoes to prepare with other ingredients included or purchase mashed potatoes from restaurants or fast-food restaurants. Did you get the point defined above? Heavily processed foods are often consumed including premade meals, frozen pizza and microwaveable dinners? Next, we will discuss the impact of sugar on the body.

Impact of sugar on the body

According to the World Health Organization (WHO), in document **TRS916** in 2003 it stated that sugar is a major cause of chronic metabolic disease and obesity; in addition, they stated that no more than 10% of the calories in the daily diet should come from sugar. In 2020 the American Heart Association reported that on average, Americans are consuming about 57 pounds of **<u>added</u>** sugar every year and the average American consumes 17 teaspoons (71.14 grams) every day. That translates into about 57 pounds of added sugar consumed each year, per person. What are the dangers of sugar to the body? Sugar is addictive. Sugar can cause the release of opioids and dopamine and can damage your immune system. Sugar robs the body of essential minerals, and it may lead to the development of cancer. The major reason to avoid consumption of sugar is because can be a detrimental to the liver. Sugar can contribute to premature aging and leads to depression, anxiety, chronic fatigue, irritability, and mood swings. In addition, sugar can increase fat storage and can affect your cholesterol. Sugar can cause insulin resistance, diabetes, and weight gain. These are some factors identified by World Health Organization's in project TRS916. The results are from studies completed throughout the world.

Keynote: For every molecule of sugar, it takes 54 molecules of magnesium to process it.

We must begin to learn the value of real food and the benefits of whole foods as well as understanding that processed foods have little or no nutritional values that our body need and require. Our bodies are considered machines that carry us from place to place as we carry out the work God has planned for us (Ephesians 2:10). An unhealthy body will make us slow, lethargic, and prone to illness and injury. Good nutrition is crucial for proper brain function and hormonal balance. Eating the right food contributes highly to our ability to think clearly and to our general quality of life. Therefore, good nutrition can help support our service for the Lord. Food is a gift from God; it is His provision. Why do whole, raw, unprocessed foods contain the most nutrition? Because they come right from God's hand.

Chapter 7: Behavioral Responsibility: Mental, Spiritual, & Physical

The Bible teaches us that our responsibility as believers is to work uncompromisingly as the Lord has gifted us and leads us in this life. We must fully understand that until the Lord returns there are souls to reach and ministries of every sort to be performed. We are responsible for our money, time, energy, talents, gifts, bodies, minds, and spirits. We should invest in nothing that does not in some way contribute to the work of the Lord. From early chapters, we learned that a small group of men obtained the monopoly and direction that healthcare should be conducted for the benefit of personal wealth gain. What do we do to change or undo the harm that has been done for so many years?

Let us analyze the key scripture for my Health ministry 1 Corinthians 6: 19-20.

Our bodies are the temple of the Holy Spirit: This principle emphasizes the importance of taking care of our physical bodies and avoiding habits that can harm them.

We are not our own: This principle reminds us that we belong to God and that our bodies are not just for our own use but are also to be used for His glory.

Holiness: This principle emphasizes the need to live a life that is holy and pleasing to God, including avoiding behaviors that can harm our physical or spiritual health is vital.

Stewardship: This principle encourages us to be good stewards of the resources and gifts that God has given us, including our physical health.

Freedom from slavery to sin: This principle emphasizes the importance of avoiding behaviors that could lead to chronic illness, such as unhealthy eating habits or substance abuse.

The power of the Holy Spirit: This principle reminds us that we have access to the power of the Holy Spirit to help us overcome chronic illness and to live a healthy and fulfilling life.

The importance of community: This principle emphasizes the importance of having a supportive community of believers who can encourage and pray for us as we deal with chronic illness.

By focusing on these biblical principles, you can be encouraged while dealing with chronic illness and have hope and healing through faith in God.

One of the key factors in obtaining good stewardship of our body and health is prioritizing our time. Use the following chart to indicate how you spend your time during a 24-hour period. Sometimes we are busy doing what is not most important to our livelihood. Evaluate how much time is spent on daily activities.

Take time to evaluate your day. In a typical 24-hour period, how many hours are spent on sleep, godly matters such as personal prayer, prayer lines, mediation, church attendance, bible reading and study. How much time is spent on worldly matters such as work, listening to the_news, or investigating what you hear concerning health alternatives. Family matters so have much time is allocated for time with spouses, children, and family chores. Remember time is like a vapor, once it's gone, we cannot get it back. So, let's use our time wisely and be intentional about not allowing anything or anyone to waste our time in an unproductive way.

Tracking Your Time

Activity	Amount of Time
Personal time	
Sleep	
Hygiene	
Exercise	
Eat	
Godly matters	
Personal prayer time	
Prayer lines	
Attend church	
Bible Reading / Study	
Worldly matters	
Work	
Listen news	
Investigate what hear	
Family matters	
Time with spouse	
Time with children	
Family chores	

How do you spend most of your time?

What areas can you change?

How much time do we listen to the worldly news versus studying God's Word?

Many times, life is about things that we have control over.

The Serenity Prayer is one of my favorites:

The Serenity Prayer
God grant me the serenity
To accept the things I cannot change;
Courage to change the things I can;
And wisdom to know the difference.

Living one day at a time;
Enjoying one moment at a time;
Accepting hardships as the pathway to peace;
Taking, as He did, this sinful world
As it is, not as I would have it;
Trusting that He will make all things right
If I surrender to His Will;
So that I may be reasonably happy in this life
And supremely happy with Him
Forever and ever in the next.

Amen

How do we accept the things we cannot change and have the courage to change things we can? Let us examine our Godly image.

As we study God's Word in Genesis 1:27– God created human beings in his own image. In the image of God, he created them. God gave us charge over the earth and everything in it. We know God regretted that he made man because of their continual sinful ways. As stated in the previous chapter, mankind is different from all other living things because we been given free will and the ability to reason. Let's now talk about being made in the image of God. We must be fully persuaded that it is our responsibility to take care of our body through education, knowledge, and faith. If we examine our body as an image of God, we have three components of our temple which is the same as the tabernacle in the Old Testament - the outer court – our body, the inner court – our soul, and the Holy of Holies – our Spirit operating according to God's will. Let's break down each area:

- **Body** – God words come through via the senses of the body. The eyes, ears, smell are avenues in which we receive information. Consider Romans 7:14-15, "The trouble is with me, for I am all too human, a slave to sin. I don't really understand myself, for I want to do what is right, but I don't do it. Instead, I do what I hate."

- **Soul** – Houses our understanding, intellect, processing skills. Romans 7:19 indicates, "I want to do what is good, but I don't. I don't want to do what is wrong, but I do it anyway."

- **Spirit** – The deepest part which is God's will. As indicated in John 14, "He is the Holy Spirit, who leads into all truth. The world cannot receive him because it isn't looking for him and doesn't recognize him. But you know him because he lives with you now and later will be in you." Other scriptural references are: Roman 8:26, 2 Corinthians 3:17, Galatians 5:22, Roman 8:27, Romans 8:11, and John 16.

3 Components of the Soul

Examine the graphic below for deeper understanding of the soul.

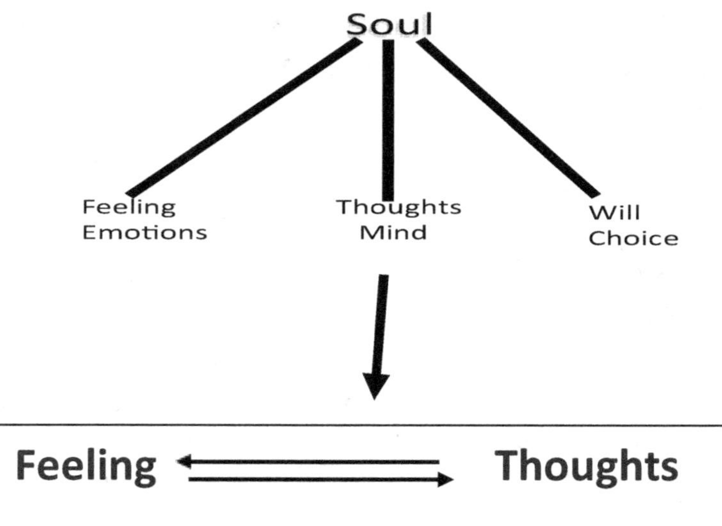

Free Will

Ability to

<u>Choose</u>

How do we get our physical body to be elevated like the tabernacle in the Old Testament scripture to the Holy of Holies? How do we obtain more energy, clearer thoughts, reduce intake of prescription medication, and allow God given food to be our medicine?

Our **free will** is a giant in our life which can be a blessing and a curse. We talk and pray about evil principalities but my brother and sister we can be our biggest enemy. Can you agree with that?

Chapter 8: Signs of Not Being Healthy

Let's discuss some signs of not being healthy. Some of the signs of not being healthy may include low or no energy, sudden loss or gain of weight, mood swings, headaches, fatigue, persistent cough, joint pain, slow healing, and swollen ankles. There are also some weird signs such as swollen legs, long ring finger, craving for ice, wrinkles in weird places, bad breath, dark urine, and black stool.

Remember your body is constantly talking to you. It is imperative that we learn what our body is trying to tell us to help avoid health issues and make the necessary lifestyle adjustments or changes.

The signs listed below are an indication of maybe some health issues:

- Low or no energy - Health-related reasons as to why you may be feeling tired may be a sign of dehydration, low iron levels, too little exercise, and too much **sugar** in the diet.

- Sudden loss of weight – Unplanned weight loss, losing 10% of body weight over 6 months may be an indication that there may be a health issue.

- Mood swings – Need to be investigated for nutritional deficiency or other psychological mental health issues.

- Headaches – Of short duration, worsen at night, early morning and don't respond to painkillers need to be checked out.

- Fatigue – Continued weakness and tiredness can be a chronic disorder or diet issue.

- Persistent cough – Accompanied with weight loss and low-grade fever should be investigated including chest x-ray.

- Slow healing – may be a sign of diabetes which can lead to slow regeneration of cells.

- Swollen ankles – May potentially be edema. When fluid accumulates in certain areas of the body, this could mean a heart issue.

- Joint pain – Accompanied with weight loss may be a sign of inflammatory disorder (Note: we will talk about inflammatory issues later).

There are some weird signs that must be mentioned here:

- Swollen legs - This is called edema, and it could be a marker of a thyroid issue (or even something more serious with your heart or kidneys)

- Long ring finger - According to a study conducted by the University of Nottingham. The research found that if your ring finger is longer than your index finger, it could be a sign that you're at a greater risk for osteoarthritis, especially in the knees.

- Craving for ice – This may mean you may have iron deficiency, as a note this is a condition can be called Pica, a disorder that causes you to crave things with no nutritional value, specifically ice (although sometimes people reach for non-food items, like dirt or paper). Interesting right?

- Wrinkles in weird places - One study published in **The Journals of Gerontology** found a different reason: high blood pressure. The research found that women with wrinkles in places typically not exposed to the sun, like the upper arms, tended to have hypertension. (Believe it or not)

- Bad breath – Even with routine mouth hygiene may be a sign of chronic bad breath can be a sign of gingivitis, a serious gum disease which can result in teeth loss if not treated.

- Dark urine - It's likely may indicate that you're dehydrated. Check your water intake daily. Recommended water intake is half of your body weight in ounces. For example, if you weigh 120 pounds then your water intake should be about 60 ounces.

- Black poop - If your stool is dark and tar like, it could be a sign of internal bleeding, often due to a stomach ulcer or other conditions.

Everyone has inflammation and typically your immune system creates the inflammation to protect the body from infection, injury, or disease:

Inflammation is classified into two main types:

- Acute inflammation – that occurs for a short (yet often severe) duration. It usually resolves in two weeks or less.

- Chronic inflammation – is slower and generally less severe but lasts longer than six weeks. It may usually not be a result of an illness or injury. This may be linked to autoimmune disorders and even prolonged stress.

Some of the signs and causes of inflammation are:

- Heat, pain, redness, swelling, and loss of other function
- Chronic and acute conditions
- Certain medications
- Exposure to irritants or foreign materials your body can't easily eliminate such as infections
- Certain foods such as Sugar
- Refined carbohydrates

- Alcohol and
- Processed meats and Trans fats

Our last topic in this chapter of not being healthy is the skin indicating that there may be a health issues. Remember in our health quiz in a previous chapter, you were asked the question what is the largest organ on our body; I hope that you named your **skin**.

Our skin covers from the top of our head to the soul of our feet. It is important to use products that are safe for our skin. The skin is incredibly resilient in its nature. Approximately every 30 days it completely regenerates. Because of this, the outer layer of skin will be gone within 7-10 days because the inner layer is growing new cells. Such insight suggests the skin is reliant on healthful living to function and look its best.

Some of the causes of unhealthy skin are:

- The most common cause of unhealthy skin is a poor diet. Diets high in refined sugars, processed meats, processed grains and dairy.

- Environmental Pollutants such as air pollutants, water pollutants, UV rays, excessive humidity, and lack of humidity

- Lack of exercise which prevents our body from carrying blood healing agents—including antioxidants. It is important to note that exercise improves the most efficient manner to deliver blood to the entire body.

- Unhealthy skin due to hygiene products are products that are free of the following ingredients:

  o **Alcohol** in your cosmetics could refer to ethanol, methanol, denatured alcohol, or ethyl alcohol and is generally found in products like perfumes, astringents, lotions, creams, and serums.

  o **Oxybenzone** is one of the most worrisome ingredients found in sunscreens that is used as a chemical filter. When absorbed by the skin, it can cause allergies and hormonal disruptions.

  o **Parabens** are synthetic compounds that are used as **preservatives** to give your products a longer shelf life. Unfortunately, very few cosmetics are free of them—they're found in everything from shampoos to shaving gels, creams to makeup and even some toothpastes.

  o **Formaldehyde** is also referred to as formalin, glyoxal and bronopol. This compound is commonly found in nail polish, eyelash glue, hair serums, foundations, and mists. It's a powerful preservative used in embalming.

  o **Talc** is related to possibly cause of cancer. Talc contains asbestos which relate to known to cause cancers in and around the lungs. Talc is usually found in dusting powders as well as powder-based makeup like eyeshadows and blushes.

- o **Phthalates** are used as binding agents, solvents, and preservatives in products like hair sprays, perfumes, deodorants, shampoos, gels, and lotions.

- o **Fragrances** are an invisibility cloak for potentially hazardous ingredients—you have no idea what's in it. Whether they're synthetic or natural, fragrances can trigger allergies, asthma, and rashes.

- o **Heavy Metals** are often found in makeup containing heavy metals like lead, mercury, and zinc. They're used in everything from lipsticks to eyeliners—and they're what gives them that metallic sheen.

Wow! In reading **all** labels we must learn to identify ingredients that are harmful to our health. We must be diligent about protecting our body according to 1Corinthians 6:19-20 and 1Corinthians 10:31 stated in the NLT "So whether you eat or drink, or whatever you do, do it all for the glory of God". We must be **fully persuaded** that we will educate, research, put into practice things that will protect and glorify our body for God's use.

Remember: You Have Free Will!!

What will you decide............?

Chapter 9: Shopping for Healthy Living

What is shopping for healthy living? There are a few steps that we must put into place to ensure that our selections are healthy for our ourselves as well as our family. Let's discuss shopping for food, cosmetics, and the environment.

Food

a. When shopping for food, focus on whole, minimally processed foods. These include fresh fruits and vegetables, whole grains, lean proteins, and healthy fats. Choose a variety of colorful fruits and vegetables to ensure you are getting a range of essential vitamins and minerals. Opt for in-season produce, as they tend to be fresher and less expensive. When buying canned or frozen produce, look for options that are packed in water or their own juice rather than syrup. Read food labels and look for products with low levels of added sugars, saturated trans fats, and sodium. Choose foods that are high in fiber, vitamins, and minerals, and limit your consumption of highly processed snacks and junk foods.

b. Look for products that are organic and non-GMO whenever possible. Note: To identify GMO fruits, God did not make anything without a seed to reproduce itself. So... seedless grapes, watermelons, lemons, etc. are all Genetic Modified Organism (GMO)meaning man genetically modified.

c. Whole grains - Choose whole grain bread, pasta, and rice instead of their refined counterparts. Look for products that have whole grain listed as the first ingredient. Try to incorporate a variety of whole grains, such as brown rice, quinoa, and barley, into your diet.

d. Lean Proteins - choose lean proteins, such as chicken, fish, turkey, and tofu, over higher-fat options like beef and pork. Look for products that are low in saturated fat and have been raised without hormones or antibiotics. Consider incorporating plant-based proteins, such as beans and legumes, into your diet.

e. Healthy fats - Choose healthy fats, such as those found in avocados, nuts, seeds, and olive oil, instead of unhealthy fats, like those found in processed snacks. Look for products that are high in monounsaturated and polyunsaturated fats, and low in saturated and trans fats. Try to limit your intake of unhealthy fats, such as those found in fried foods, processed snacks, and hydrogenated oils.

f. Dairy - Choose low-fat or fat-free dairy products, such as milk, cheese, and yogurt, to limit your saturated fat intake. Look for products that are high in calcium and other essential vitamins and minerals. Consider trying dairy-free alternatives, such as almond milk or soy milk, if you are lactose intolerant or have a milk allergy.

g. Beverages - choose water, unsweetened tea, and low-fat milk as your primary beverages. Limit your intake of sugary drinks, such as soda and fruit juice, as these can be high in added sugars and calories. Consider drinking herbal teas or infused water for a flavorful and low-calorie alternative.

Note: when selecting low fat or fat free products look for sugar or other sugar ingredients added. By following these guidelines, you can make healthier food choices and build a balanced, nutritious diet.

Cosmetics

a. When shopping for cosmetics, look for products that are free of harmful chemicals, such as parabens, phthalates, and sodium lauryl sulfate.

b. Choose cosmetics that are cruelty-free and have not been tested on animals.

c. Read the ingredient list and choose products that are made with natural, plant-based ingredients.

d. Look for cosmetics that are free of synthetic fragrances, as these can be irritants for some people.

Environment

a. When shopping for household and personal care products, look for items that are environmentally friendly and made with non-toxic ingredients.

b. Choose products that are biodegradable and made from renewable resources.

c. Avoid products that contain harmful chemicals, such as chlorine, ammonia, and phthalates. (Also check the list above of harmful ingredients.)

d. Look for products that are Energy Star certified, as these products are energy-efficient and have a lower impact on the environment.

Remember, when shopping for food, cosmetics, and environment products, it's important to consider your personal health and environmental impact. Look for products that are safe and sustainable and be an informed and conscious consumer.

Also, remember that Investing in your wellbeing and your family is pleasing to God in terms of honoring our body.

Chapter 10: Keys to Run your Healthy Race

Be good stewards of your body by being fully persuaded committed to a healthier life style. Consider your ways and realize that you have a responsibility to your health. Of course, no matter what our physical condition is, we can serve the Lord. But the healthier we are physically, the more effectively we can serve God. Stewarding your body well isn't about becoming a certain size. It's not about obsessing over portion sizes and calories. It's about taking the best care of yourself possible. If God wanted us all to be the same size and shape – He'd have made us that way. Guess what – God wants you to be the size and shape He created you to be. When you steward your body well and care for it in a way that glorifies God – that's all that matters.

Let's look at some scriptures:

1 Corinthians 3:16-19, Don't you realize that all of you together are the temple of God and that the Spirit of God lives in you? God will destroy anyone who destroys this temple. For God's temple is holy, and you are that temple. Stop deceiving yourselves. If you think you are

wise by this world's standards, you need to become a fool to be truly wise. For the wisdom of this world is foolishness to God. As the Scriptures says, "He traps the wise in the snare of their own cleverness."

God tells us in 1 Corinthians 6: 19-20, that our body is the temple of the Holy Spirit which is an honor in stewardship of our physical body. The Word of God further states that the world hates us as they hated him. John 15:18-19, Satan is constantly looking to deceive and conquer. Do we believe because we are Christians that the world gives us favor and look out for our good? We are sadly mistaken if we do.

1 John 2: 15-17, Do not love this world nor the things it offers you, for when you love the world, you do not have the love of the Father in you. 1 John 2:16-17, For the world offers only a craving for physical pleasure, a craving for everything we see, and pride in our achievements and possessions. These are not from the Father but are from this world. And this world is fading away, along with everything that people crave. But anyone who does what pleases God will live forever.

We studied how the world has changed the medical community starting with the Flexner Report and somewhat limited our medical choices. We have further studied that there is a trust of worldly companies working together to control our health choices, food choices, and resolutions for health issues. Is the world making a mockery of the body of Christ? We have been given instructions on the foods we should eat regarding the foods we should from the five food groups, and we will produce healthy bodies. If this is true, why is God's creation so sick in America?

Look at the Covid Pandemic in 2019-2020, our country pays more for health insurance than all other countries combined. Yet, the question remains, why did America have the highest cases of covid infection and the highest death rate? The handwriting is on the wall we must change our lifestyle habits and more importantly change the lifestyle behavior for our children and generation to come.

If we believe and operate in it. We have a radically supernatural lifestyle. We have dominion over the natural and the supernatural. We are surrounded by and led by the ever-present voice of the Trinity, the Spirit of the Lord, the Spirit of Wisdom and Revelation, the Spirit of Counsel, the Spirit of Understanding, the Spirit of Knowledge, the Spirit of Might, and the Spirit of Fear of the Lord. In addition, the Divine appointment, Divine health, Divine relationships, Divine abundance, and Divine Life are all at our fingertips if we only tap into what are our God given resources.

In the Book of Haggai in the Bible, the Israelites were free from exile, they started building their house and neglecting the house of God as a result the house of God was left in ruin. God sent prophet Haggai with a message:

In KJV translation, Haggai 1: 5, 7 "Consider your ways". In NLT it is written as "Look at what's happening to you!"

What is our Christian responsibility? Since our body is the house of God that has been created by God according to His Word in 1 Corinthians 6:19-20. The question to ask: What value do you place on your physical body?

Food for thought:

- Of course, no matter what our physical condition, we can serve the Lord. But the healthier we are physically, the more effectively we can do that.

- Honor God with food: God created men and women in His image, blessed them and charged them with filling the earth and subduing it (Gen. 1:28-29). He then made food as a provision for His creatures. He gifted us with fuel to sustain, nourish and energize our bodies for worship and witness. We fuel our bodies for the glory of God and good of others. The Bible reminds us that our freedom is not "to indulge the flesh" but instead to "serve one another humbly in love" (Gal. 5:13, NIV). The Bible reminds us that we are not our own but that we have been bought with a price and are to glorify God in our body (1 Cor. 6:19-20). Yet the Bible also reminds us to eat and drink with enjoyment because these are from God's hand (Ecclesiastes 2:24, 9:7).

- Healthy living begins with healthy thinking. Discipline is the road to the good life.

- "The road to life is a disciplined life; ignore correction and you're lost for good" (Proverbs 10:17, MSG).

In 1 Corinthians 9:24-27 the Word states:

"Don't you realize that in a race everyone runs, but only one person gets the prize? So run to win! All athletes are disciplined in their training. They do it to win a prize that will fade away, but we do it for an eternal prize. So, I run with purpose in every step. I am not just shadowboxing. I discipline my body like an athlete, training it to do what it should. Otherwise, I fear that after preaching to others I myself might be disqualified."

What do you believe? In this world that belief from a scientific point of view (this world just evolved by nature). Once the body breaks down it cannot change, and we must treat the body's symptoms, or do you believe that God has magnificently made everything and His magnificent creation is man? Do you believe that God created the human body to repair itself? Once we have the knowledge of what we should take out of our diet and what we should give our body to support its function, our bodies can function at its maximum capacity.

The Bibles tell us in Psalms 8: 4-6, "What is mankind that you are mindful of them, human beings that you care for them? You have made them a little lower than the angels and crowned them with glory and honor.

You made them rulers over the works of your hands; you put everything under their feet." (KJV)

If this is God's thought about us as human beings, what are our thoughts about ourselves? Believe it or not that our thoughts do create our reality. Our thoughts should be always positive minded. Negative patterns of thinking are dangerous because it undermines God's Word, the truth, and our faith. Just as in earlier chapter we were told that "We are what we eat". The same holds true about our thoughts. We become what we think about ourselves. Negative thoughts steal our energy; make us weak; give life to negative imaginations to make them a reality. Our mind does not really know the truth and our mind responds to what we tell it. In Philippians 4:8 (KJV), God tells us what kind of thoughts to think about ourselves: "Finally, brethren, whatever is true, whatever is noble, whatever is right, whatever is pure, whatever is lovely, whatever is admirable – if anything is excellent or praiseworthy – think about such things." The conclusion is that when you think positive thoughts about yourself, the thoughts will grow and become a stronghold in your mind and eventually your reality.

The Bible teaches us that our responsibility as believer is to work uncompromisingly as the Lord has gifted us and leads us in this life. We must fully understand that until the Lord returns there are souls to reach and ministries of every sort to be performed. We are responsible for our money, time, energy, talents, gifts, **bodies**, minds, and spirits, and we should invest in nothing that does not in some way contribute to the work of the Lord.

In Jeremiah 17:5-10, This is what the Lord says: "Cursed are those who put their trust in mere humans, who rely on human strength and turn their hearts away from the Lord. They are like stunted shrubs in the desert, with no hope for the future. They will live in the barren wilderness, in an uninhabited salty land. But blessed are those who trust in the Lord and have made the Lord their hope and confidence. They are like trees planted along a riverbank, with roots that reach deep into the water. Such trees are not bothered by the heat or worried by long months of drought. Their leaves stay green, and they never stop producing fruit. The human heart is the most deceitful of all things, and desperately wicked. Who really knows how bad it is? But I, the Lord, search all hearts and examine secret motives. I give all people their due rewards, according to what their actions deserve." Wow, we do not know any explanation about this scripture. I personally want to have a heart and mind like a blessed one. What about you?

Let us examine ourselves.

"Because we have these promises, dear friends, let us cleanse ourselves from everything that can defile our body or spirit. And let us work toward complete holiness because we fear God." 2 Corinthians 7:1

In Acts 17:30-31, God overlooked people's ignorance about these things in earlier times, but now he commands everyone everywhere to repent of theirs sins and turn to him. For he has set a day for judging the world with justice by the man he has appointed, and he proved to everyone who this is by raising him from the dead.

I suggest the following recommended book resources:

- Dr. Joel Wallach, ND "Hell's kitchen"
- William Davis, MD cardiologist "Wheat Belly"
- David Permutter, MD Neurologist "Grain Brain"
- Rex Steven Spikes, "Life on Your Terms – Create the Life You Want!"

In Summary:
We need to realize that we are the reason why we have health issues whether we were aware or not or didn't think we needed to know anything about our body or are dependent on someone else to take charge of our health. Now, that you have been provided basic information, what changes are you willing to make for you and your family? Will you evaluate what you are eating? Will you begin to read food labels, cosmetics labels, and environmental labels? Will you maintain knowledge of the various harmful ingredients?

We are responsible for being healthy and keeping our loved ones healthy. One of my favorite anecdotes is as follows:

You have a beautiful house with beautiful lawns and flowers, However, in the front yard is a giant tree that is an eye sore. Besides that it secretes a sap that sticks to your sidewalk, and it has damaged some of your landscape. You decide to get rid of the tree, so you get your saw and go to the tree and cut off one of the branches. You go back into the house believing that you have taken care of that problem. However the branch grows back stronger.   So what's the moral of the anecdote? Cutting off a branch is not enough. We must get to the root of the problem. A surface solution can produce lifelong problems but getting to root of the problem can produce freedom, health and wealth.

Here is a devotion that I saw from Lion Bites Global alliance that I believe that we all can receive and mediate on the message.

A Holy Place

You exist where heaven meets earth. You are the home of the Holy Spirit. You are a Holy Place!

God is calling your self-perspective into right alignment with how He sees you. For out of all the places that God could live, He chose you. Marvel at this! God's breath is in your lungs, God's Spirit is in your heart, God's seal is upon you. Every part of your body bears the fingerprints of the Lord Almighty. How beautiful is the work of his hands.

It is time to stop slandering the temple where the Holy Spirit of God dwells. It's time to stop speaking negativity over yourself. Take time today to thank God for your body, where he so richly lives. Marvel at how God thinks you are so wonderful; he has made you, his home. Delight in being a carrier of God himself. Bless your body as a holy place for the Spirit of God and call yourself beautiful. For child of God, you are indeed a beautiful holy place.

Activation: *Speak life over yourself today! Ask Holy Spirit to lead you through declarations of life and love, speaking to them aloud over yourself.*

1 Corinthians 6:19 (NIV) Or do you not know that your body is a temple of the Holy Spirit who is in you, whom you have from God, and that you are not your own?

1 John 3:1 (TPT) Look with wonder at the depth of the Father's marvelous love that he has lavished upon us! He has called us and made us his very own beloved children.

What do you believe? Will you investigate and invest into your physical body as the temple of the Holy spirit? Because you have **free will!!**

Remember: Nothing changes until you change. Everything changes when you change.

79

Appendix 1

Answer to Exercise 1

1. Genetic Modified Organism

2. Tooth enamel

3. False Glue-like protein. The body do not know how to process the new gluten.

4. Skin

5. Keratin, a type of protein that's a basic component of hair, skin, and nails.

6. False: According to U.S. Senate document #264 back in 1936, our farmlands have been depleted of essential minerals